Flu:
Staying and Keeping Your Family Safe

THIS HOLIDAY SEASON

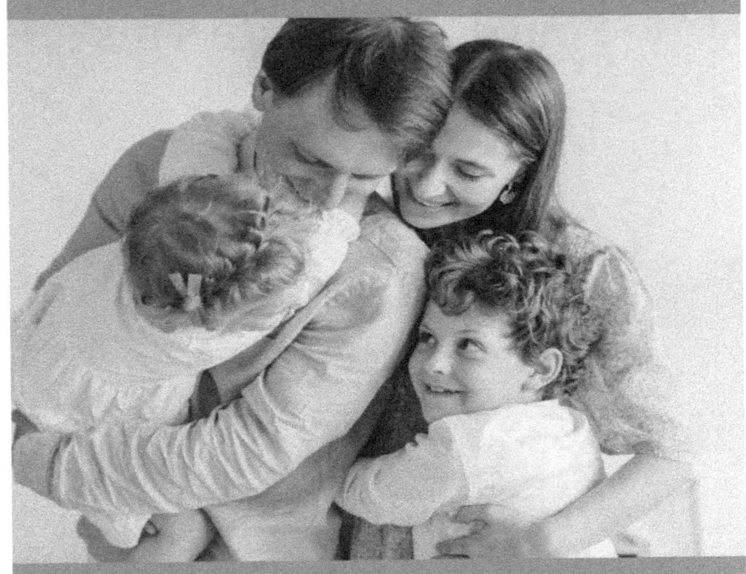

RACHAEL PHILIP

Flu:

Staying And Keeping

Your Family Safe This

Holiday Season

By

Rachael Philip

Table of Contents

Introduction

What is the flu?

Flu (influenza) is an infection of the nose, throat, and lungs, part of the respiratory system.

Influenza is commonly called the flu, but it's not the same as stomach "flu" viruses that cause diarrhea and vomiting.

Most people with the flu get better on their own, but the flu is a virus that can make you feel really sick and very uncomfortable.

It's important to know the symptoms and to get help if you think you might have the flu.

There are things you can do to feel better, and there are medicines that can help too.

The flu is different from a cold and can be much more serious.

Flu symptoms come on suddenly and can include fever, chills, body aches, headache, coughing, and feeling very tired.

You might also have a sore throat, runny nose, nausea, and vomiting. For the most part, the flu is unpleasant but not dangerous.

However, some people are more vulnerable to serious flu complications, like pneumonia.

These include pregnant women, young children, older adults, and people with chronic medical conditions like heart disease or diabetes.

The best way to avoid getting the flu in the first place is to take care of yourself.

This includes frequently washing your hands, avoiding sick people, and getting a flu shot every year.

Eating well and getting enough rest can also go a long way.

Flu season typically lasts from October to May in the United States, with peak activity occurring between December and February.

So now is a great time to ensure you and your family have your vaccinations up to date!

If you get the flu, you must stay home and rest until you are no longer contagious.

Chapter One: What is the flu, and how does it spread?

The flu (influenza) is an infection of the nose, throat, and lungs.

It is a virus that can make you feel sick and is more contagious than the common cold.

The best prevention for flu is to get vaccinated each year.

Fever is exceptionally uncomfortable and must be avoided at all costs.

In addition, it is crucial to stay hydrated and rest when you have a fever.

It's a virus that spreads quickly from person to person.

Most experts believe that flu viruses spread primarily through droplets produced when people with the flu cough, sneeze or talk.

These droplets can land in the mouths or noses of nearby people (usually within 6 feet) or be inhaled into the lungs.

The flu virus is most commonly transmitted from person to person through the air we breathe, but it is also transferred through the surfaces we touch.

Keep in mind that there are simple steps you can take to help protect yourself and your loved ones from the

flu this season.

Chapter Two: Why it spreads easier during the winter months

The flu is a more serious illness than the common cold, and it can be fatal in some cases.

Like every other contagious disease, it can occur at any time but has seasons when it spikes.

Top University doctors say the winter season is when we have the most respiratory infections. They explain further that respiratory infections spread more easily and quickly for two reasons.

First, we spend more time in enclosed spaces, resulting in more prolonged face-to-face contact.

The second reason is related to humidity.

We're usually 3 to 6 feet apart when we pass viruses from one person to another — the so-called 'breathing zone.'

When we have low humidity, such as in the winter, there is little moisture surrounding the virus to allow it to evaporate, so the virus remains in the air for an extended period of time.

If a person is close enough to someone who has the virus, they will be able to breathe it in.

Perhaps you may have heard that getting caught in the rain and staying in wet clothes can cause a cold.

Experts suggest this is a myth.

They proffer that this school of thought was initiated to people indoors during bad weather.

Limited knowledge of viruses and their function may be why people associate being cold with getting the flu.

Besides, anyone would remember when they got sick and where they were when it happened, but people tend to forget the times they were actually cold and wet but didn't get sick just because they did not get sick.

It's understandable that before anyone knew about germs, the cold and shiver one feels when wet would be similar to the cold and shiver of fever and illness.

This makes it easy to believe one is related to the other.

It also stands to reason that because viruses thrive in cold weather, we get sick more efficiently when the weather is cold.

We now know that viruses cause colds, and viruses or bacteria cause pneumonia, so you can only get sick if exposed to these germs, regardless of the weather.

According to the Centers for Disease
Control and Prevention (CDC) Trusted
Source, millions of people get the
common cold each year, with the
average adult getting two to three
colds.

Children usually get even more.

Most people get colds in the winter or
spring, but they can occur at any time
of year.

Chapter Three: When are the most vulnerable times to catch and spread the flu?

As has already been stated, seasonal influenza is present all year in the United States, but it is most prevalent in the fall and winter.

Some argue that the term influenza is derived from the Italian phrase "influenza di freddo," which means "cold influence."

Although experts agree that colder weather facilitates the spread of the flu virus, they also point to other factors as contributing to the spike in influenza cases during the winter and fall.

In many cases, if the right circumstances are present, viruses can survive in colder temperatures if the right circumstances are present.

Temperature and humidity play a major role, but they don't explain everything, since human activity and choices also expose us to viruses and bacteria.

In temperate zones, the flu season usually does coincide with colder months.

But in the tropics, flu is often associated with the rainy seasons and may occur year-round or show both winter months and summer months peaks.

Additionally, a lot of our pandemics, like the one in 2009, seem to start in the late spring and early summer after the official flu season has ended.

The immune system may also be impacted by inadequate sunlight exposure during the colder months, but this has not been verified.

How sunlight influences all of this has yet to be well known.

However, it is well known that the sun's ultraviolet light serves as a powerful decontaminant.

In the past, before the discovery of antibiotics, exposing tuberculosis patients to the sun aided in their recovery.

Chapter Four: What are the flu symptoms, and how can you tell if you have it or not?

Sudden onset of illness is typical, and

the flu is frequently to blame.

A cold is not caused by a virus like the

flu or a respiratory illness.

Knowing the signs of the flu is

essential for contacting medical

assistance if needed.

The following advice can help you lower your risk of influenza-related death.

Flu symptoms include fever, chills, body aches, headache, coughing, and extreme exhaustion. They also appear suddenly.

In addition, you could experience nausea and vomiting, a runny nose, and a sore throat.

Some people are particularly vulnerable to the flu's serious side effects.

These people include expectant mothers, young children, senior citizens, and those who suffer from long-term illnesses like diabetes or heart disease.

Washing your hands often, staying away from sick people, and getting a flu vaccine every year are strong preventive measures.

Consume fiber-rich, balanced diets and rest when the flu is present.

The most prevalent and early sign of the flu is a headache.

It's crucial to get lots of liquids in you and get plenty of rest if you have a headache.

Make an appointment with your doctor if your headache is severe or lasts for more than a few days, even when you've taken relief medicines.

The worst of your symptoms will pass once you reach day 3, which will happen around day 2 or 3.

Your immune system is working hard to contain the infection during this stage, so you are less contagious since you are still in the contagious phase of the flu.

How do I know if my flu is getting better?

The fever will begin to recede, and you will start to gain strength and become aware of your environment. You will also notice that you are sweating more, and this is a good sign.

A sudden increase in appetite is also a good sign to look out for.

Chapter Five: How can you prevent the flu from spreading to others, and what should you do if you get sick yourself?

The flu is a more severe illness than the common cold and can sometimes be deadly.

Make sure you get your shots every year.

One of the best ways to stop the flu from spreading is by regularly washing your hands.

Additionally, you should keep your distance from sick people and clean frequently touched surfaces.

If you do end up getting the flu, it's crucial to stay out of public places and limit contact with family and loved ones until you are no longer contagious.

Regardless of whether you feel sick or not, never touch your face.

You must receive an annual flu shot if you are a pregnant woman, a child, an adult, or have a chronic health condition. In other words, everyone needs a picture.

In addition to helping you stay healthy, the vaccine can lower your risk of developing serious side effects if you contract the flu.

Flu activity has been reported in the United States this season in a moderately high volume.

You still have time to get vaccinated, so ask your doctor if you and your family are up to date on your shots.

These easy precautions can assist in defending you and those close to you from the flu this season.

Chapter Six: Can the flu be deadly, and what are some steps to take to reduce the risk of death from influenza?

Yes, the flu can sometimes be fatal, especially for high-risk groups like expectant mothers, young children, older adults, and those with a history of chronic illness.

If you do end up getting the flu, it's crucial to see your doctor as soon as possible so that you can begin taking antiviral medication.

These medications can lessen the severity of your illness and help shorten its duration.

Additionally, it's crucial to avoid spreading the flu to others by staying home from work or school until you are no longer contagious.

If you are at high risk for complications from the flu, be sure to talk to your doctor about what you can do to protect yourself.

Taking simple measures can help reduce your risk of getting sick or spreading the flu to others.

Frequently washing your hands in soapy water for at least 20 seconds and avoiding touching your face, eyes, nose, or mouth with unwashed hands are the best ways to prevent getting a cold.

Additionally, you should make an effort to stay away from people who are coughing or sneezing up close and frequently clean frequently touched surfaces in your home, such as doorknobs and other handles.

When going outside, be sure to dress warmly and comfortably. You should also maintain healthy eating and exercise habits and avoid overexerting yourself.

Chapter Seven: Best Foods To Eat When You Get The Flu

Get as much fluid into your body as you can before anything else.

Your body requires additional fluids when you have the flu or any other illness that raises your temperature.

Stay hydrated because your body needs fluids more than it needs food when you have a disease because it is so easy to become dehydrated.

Water, electrolyte-rich beverages, broths, and herbal tea are all suitable alternatives.

Just stay away from sugary drinks and caffeinated drinks like soda and coffee, as they could further dehydrate you.

Your body needs more nutrients than usual when you're ill because your immune system serves as your body's defense against invaders like the flu, so it's important to nourish it properly by healing and refilling lost nutrients.

Best Foods To Eat When Sick With The Flu

Broth

Broth is high in minerals and antioxidants, and it helps to keep you hydrated.

It's also warm and cozy, which will help to soothe your sore throat and clear your stuffy nose.

If you're reading this before the flu hits, make your own broth — whether it's a vegetarian version or an electrolyte-rich bone broth — to keep in the freezer in case it comes in handy.

Although making it yourself is the best option, you can also buy it from the grocery store or order it from a local restaurant if you're too sick to prepare it.

Soup with chicken

By adding chicken and nutritious vegetables to your broth, you can boost the protein and iron content and help your body fight the flu.

The warmth of the liquid will soothe your sore throat whether you choose matzah ball soup, lentil dal, or plain old canned chicken noodle soup.

According to one study, the nutrients in chicken soup reduce inflammation and improve your immune system's response to disease.

Popsicles on ice

Warm beverages are more likely to relieve a sore throat than cold ones, but if you want to try something different (and stay hydrated), an ice treat may help cool down the inflamed tissue.

Just make sure they're all-natural and don't have any added sugars, and you can even make your own!

Vitamin C-rich fruits and vegetables

Vitamin C is linked to a stronger immune system and may help with cold and flu symptoms.

Examples of fruits and vegetables packed with Vitamin C

Oranges and grapefruits are examples of citrus fruits

Broccoli

The Brussels sprouts

Cantaloupe

Kiwi

Peppers

Potatoes

Strawberries

Tomatoes

Greens with leaves

Salads may not seem like comfort
food, but greens like spinach, kale,
and cabbage are high in vitamin C and

iron, which helps reduce inflammation and help you feel better sooner.

If the thought of eating a salad makes you sick, try adding a leafy green to your chicken soup or other hearty stew to reap the benefits in a more flu-friendly form.

Juice from fruits or vegetables

Bring on the orange juice! Whole fruits and vegetables are usually preferable, but when you're sick, you can't eat much.

In a pinch, drink natural fruit or vegetable juice to supplement your diet.

Tea with herbs

Hot tea can soothe a sore throat, and the steam can help clear a stuffy nose.

Add some honey for an extra calming boost.

It has been shown to promote sleep and reduce nighttime coughing in sick children (but not to children under the age of 12 months).

Garlic

Consuming raw garlic may boost your immune system, according to research.

Raw garlic is more beneficial than cooked garlic or garlic supplements.

You can also use it in hot tea with a little honey to mask the strong fragrance and improve the taste.

Calming spices

Ginger, cayenne pepper, and turmeric are also associated with a variety of warm, comforting dishes, each with its own set of health benefits.

Make use of comfort foods

When you're sick with the flu, you may not want to eat much, so eat whatever sounds best at the time and make sure you continue to put some

nutrients in you no matter how you

feel about it.

Everything tastes strange when you're

sick, and you frequently lose your

appetite.

Choosing meals that make you happy

may make you feel better while also

providing your body with the calories

and nutrients it needs.

The BRAT diet

BRAT stands for bananas, (white) rice, apples, and toast, and it refers to low-fiber meals that will help you feel better.

These simple meals are easy to digest and are frequently recommended when someone is ill.

This diet, however, is associated with stomach flu and not influenza.

It may still be a good option when you

have no appetite for any other thing.

The BRAT Diet is low in vitamins and

minerals, but it's gentle on your body,

so if that's what you want, go for it.

Chapter Eight: Food To Avoid When You Have The Flu

Nothing seems to make you feel better (or worse) when you have the flu.

However, assistance may arrive from an unexpected source.

Surprisingly, some foods may worsen — or improve — your flu symptoms without your knowledge.

Eating can be difficult because flu symptoms can cause nausea or stomach cramps.

When food is consumed too quickly, nausea can reduce the desire to eat, and gastrointestinal symptoms such as vomiting and diarrhea can occur.

Eating nutrient-dense foods is beneficial regardless of illness, but it is especially important when you have a fever.

However, not all food is created equal; while comfort foods may be what you crave when you aren't feeling well, they're not necessarily going to make you feel better.

Avoid these four foods when you have the flu:

Caffeinated drinks and alcohol

When you have a fever, you should be cautious of dehydration due to increased sweating and high temperatures.

Caffeine and alcohol can aggravate your symptoms (especially stomach-related symptoms), so stay hydrated by avoiding them.

Greasy foods

Foods that are difficult to digest and hard on your digestive system should be avoided.

Saturated fats, as well as fried and greasy foods, should be avoided or consumed in moderation.

Hard-to-digest grains

Because the flu can cause stomach upset, it is best to stick to easy-to-digest foods like simple/refined carbohydrates.

Foods that are easy on the stomach, such as dry saltine crackers, toast, and pretzels, are more likely to be tolerated when you have the flu.

Sugary food or drinks

While you may believe that drinking vitamin-c-rich fruit juices is the best thing to do when you're sick, the majority of these options aren't nutritionally dense and can actually aggravate your immune system.

Stay hydrated by drinking water and other clear liquids.

Chapter Nine: What To Avoid When You Have The Flu

If you get the flu, regular flu shots will not help you recover, but there are prescription antiviral drugs that can help with influenza when nothing else does.

Antibiotics can also cause yeast infections, upset stomachs, and diarrhea as side effects.

Antibiotics are now being shown to have long-term effects on the bacteria in your gut.

In addition to being completely ineffective at treating the flu, overuse of antibiotics can lead to resistance. Then when they need them, the antibiotics fail.

Don't medicate with a hot toddy

You may have been told that a hot, boozy drink eased the flu's symptoms, but that's not right.

While alcohol soothes raw throats and quiets coughs (it's a cough suppressant, which is why it's in over-the-counter cough medications), it also causes dehydration, which compounds the dehydration caused by the flu.

Drowsiness is caused by excessive alcohol consumption, as is drowsiness caused by some over-the-counter cold medications.

Combining cold medicine and alcohol can be hazardous, so avoid it.

Skip the nasal spray

Some people use decongestant nasal sprays to relieve the pain of clogged noses, but they may cause more harm than good.

Do not use nasal sprays for more than three days; the more frequently they are used, the less likely they are to work.

Once the effect wears off, you will experience rebound swelling, which means you will need to use nasal sprays again and again.

Nasal congestion often signals a cold, not the flu.

The Centers for Disease Control and Prevention recommends that children under 2, people over 65, and people with chronic conditions receive antiviral medication for the flu to avoid complications.

Don't go to work

They are going to work or school while sick means infecting others.

Furthermore, because there are

multiple strains of flu, people are at

risk of contracting it.

Chapter Ten: Boosting Your Immunity this Fall and Winter Season

There are things you can do to help give your immune system what it needs in order to function optimally when required, but none of these require the use of a supplement.

Here are five scientifically proven methods for developing and maintaining a strong, healthy immune system:

1. Keep up to date on recommended vaccines.

Having a strong immune system means taking advantage of the best advantage we have.

Your immune system is intelligent, but vaccines train it to be even more so, teaching it how to recognize and combat disease-causing illnesses.

Vaccination is far safer for your immune system than infection with these dangerous germs.

It's always a good idea to stay current on recommended vaccinations, especially your COVID-19 vaccine or booster and your annual flu shot.

2. Follow a healthy diet

A healthy diet, like most things in your body, is essential for a strong immune system.

This includes eating plenty of vegetables, fruits, legumes, and grains.

A healthy diet can help ensure you get enough of the micronutrients that play a role in immune system maintenance, in addition to providing your immune system with the energy it requires.

- Vitamin B6, can be found in chicken, salmon, tuna, bananas, green vegetables, and potatoes (with skin).
- Citrus fruits, such as oranges and strawberries, as well as tomatoes, broccoli, and spinach, contain vitamin C.

⊠ Almonds, sunflower and safflower oil, sunflower seeds, peanut butter, and spinach all contain vitamin E.

Because experts believe that your body absorbs vitamins more efficiently from dietary sources rather than supplements, eating a well-balanced diet is the best way to support your immune system.

3. Regular physical activity

Physical activity isn't just for muscle building and stress relief; it's also an important part of staying healthy and supporting a healthy lifestyle.

Exercise may improve immune function by increasing overall circulation, allowing immune cells and other infection-fighting molecules to travel more easily throughout your body.

In fact, studies have shown that even 30 minutes of moderate-to-vigorous exercise per day can help stimulate your immune system.

This means that it's critical to prioritize staying active and getting regular exercise.

4. Always drink water

Water serves many functions in your body, including immune system support.

Lymph is a fluid in your circulatory system that carries important infection-fighting immune cells around your body.

Dehydration slows the movement of lymph, which can result in an impaired immune system.

Even if you aren't exercising or sweating, you are constantly losing water through your breath, urine, and bowel movements.

To help your immune system, make sure you're replacing the water you lose with usable water.

5. Get enough sleep

Sleep does not appear to be an active process, but there are many

important things going on in your
body when you are not awake.

Important infection-fighting
molecules, for example, are produced
while you sleep.

According to studies, people who do
not get enough quality sleep are more
likely to become ill.

To give your immune system the best
chance of fighting infection and

illness, it's critical to understand how much sleep you should get each night and what to do if your rest is suffering.

6. *Reduce your stress levels*

It's critical to understand how stress affects your health, whether it comes on suddenly or gradually.

When you are under prolonged stress, your body responds by triggering what is known as a stress response.

It is intended to assist you in dealing with stressful situations that may arise.

Unfortunately, this response suppresses your immune system, increasing your likelihood of infection or illness.

Stress is different for everyone, and how we relieve it is, too.

Given the impact it can have on your health, it's critical to understand how to recognize stress.

You should also become acquainted with the activities that help you reduce stress, whether they are deep breathing, meditation, prayer, or exercise.

Chapter Eleven: Where can I get more information about the flu, including contact information for local vaccination clinics?

The Centers for Disease Control and Prevention (CDC) has a wealth of information on the flu, including how to stay healthy and what to do if you become ill.

The CDC website also has resources for vaccination clinics in your area.

Getting vaccinated each year is the best way to protect yourself and your family from the flu.

Many doctors' offices, pharmacies, and health departments offer flu vaccines for free or at a low cost.

You can also find out if there are any vaccination clinics in your area by visiting the CDC website or contacting the local health department.

Protecting yourself and your loved ones from the flu is a critical part of staying healthy during flu season.

Chapter Twelve: Flu Home Remedies

There are several home remedies that can help relieve flu symptoms, some of which are as follows:

-Sleep and drink plenty of fluids

-Using over-the-counter medications to reduce fever and pain, such as ibuprofen or acetaminophen

-Use a humidifier to help relieve congestion.

-Drinking hot beverages such as tea or chicken soup

-Consuming popsicles or other frozen desserts

-Using a warm compress on your chest or back

If you are experiencing severe symptoms, you should see a doctor as soon as possible.

Home remedies can help relieve mild to moderate flu symptoms but will not cure the virus.

If you are at high risk of complications, you must seek medical attention immediately.

Regardless of your risk, you should consult a doctor if your symptoms do not improve or worsen.